How to Look Younger

Health and beauty advice for women who
want to keep looking and feeling fabulous

Susan Lomas

Susan Lomas

ISBN-13: 978-1492959250
ISBN-10: 1492959251

Published by SusanLomas.com
Version CS1.0

Table of Contents

Susan Lomas

Foreword

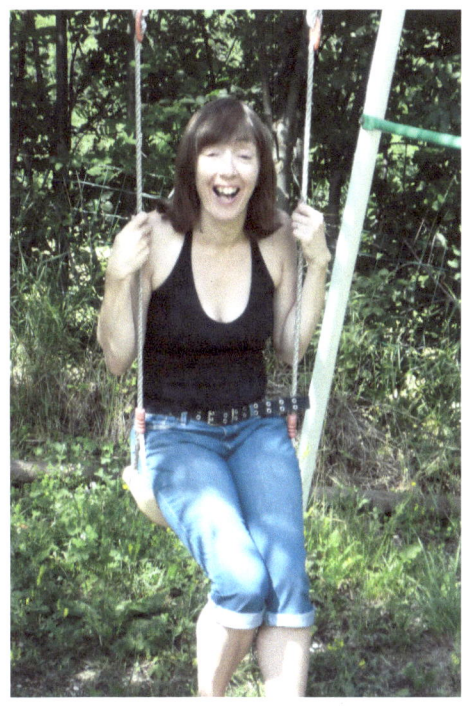

This book contains realistic advice for real women. The idea was actually suggested to me by an ex-boyfriend who I happened to "bump into" on Facebook after many years. He commented that I didn't look much older than when we dated back in the 1980s and also said

"Hey, if you like writing books why not write a book about looking young?"

Who will enjoy reading this book? I think that there is useful wisdom in here for women of all ages. Those in their twenties and thirties will find practical information about how to build a strong, womanly body by eating and exercising well. I also discuss the ageing effects of too much sun exposure and smoking on the skin.

For women in their forties, fifties and beyond there are tips on how to dress and look after your skin and hair so that you continue to look and feel fabulous.

Throughout the book I emphasise the natural ways to keep looking young and feeling young. However I felt it would be interesting to include a section about cosmetic surgery as a contrast.

I wrote this book when I was 49 years old but I am lucky enough to have both younger and older female friends (including some in their late fifties or sixties who are fabulous, positive people). I have included more than a few snippets of wisdom from enjoyable conversations we've had when out walking, or having a coffee together.

My message is largely "Everything in moderation, drink plenty of water and don't forget to get a good night's sleep."

Happy reading!

Body shape

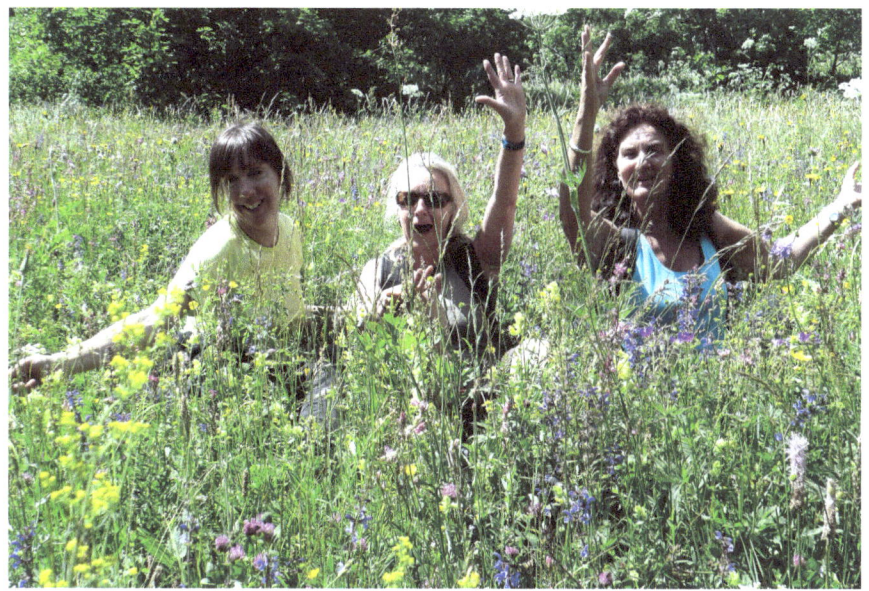

Are you an ectomorph, mesomorph or an endomorph?

We all inherit particular physical characteristics from our biological parents, such as height and bone structure. If you wish to keep looking young and feeling healthy you need to learn to work with what you've got, to a certain extent. If you eat and drink healthily without excessive dieting or bingeing you should instinctively be aware of what weight you feel comfortable at. Thank goodness that early twenty-first century role models such as Beyoncé, Shakira and Jennifer Lopez celebrate their womanly curves.

Tall, slim people, with long narrow muscles are often referred to as ectomorphs. They are fortunate in many ways because they can eat well and exercise accordingly. They find it hard to put on weight and gain muscle. Traditionally fashion designers have used ectomorph women as catwalk or runway models. If ectomorph women don't keep enough weight on as they get older they can end up looking slightly too thin, especially around the neck and face.

3

Mesomorphs have an athletic build. They are strong, often with broader shoulders than ectomorphs. Mesomorph women sometimes have to take care not to build their bodies too much when they exercise, choosing routines and a diet that encourage a feminine softness as well as strength.

Many people feel that a healthy, toned endomorph body is the most feminine shape of all. Endomorphs are usually short and tend towards a stockier build. They have a rounded physique and their muscles are not so well defined. They also have a slow metabolism and should try to eat a light diet, but with plenty of protein, vegetables, fruit and salad. However, on the plus side, a toned, fit, confident endomorph woman, such as Beyoncé, Marilyn Monroe or Scarlett Johansson, can look fabulous wearing swimsuits or very revealing outfits.

You are what you eat

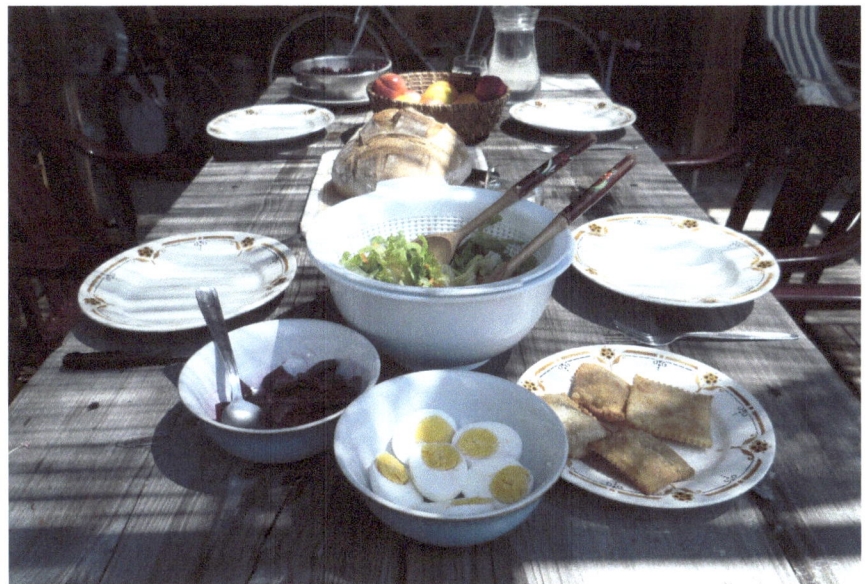

A midday meal with protein, salad, fruit and carbohydrates

It sometimes seems unfair that when we are young some of us can eat absolutely anything and not put on weight! I have to declare that I was one of those annoying individuals. However although I remain slim overall I have noticed that as I approach fifty (and after giving birth to two children) my waistline needs more watching than before. Your body mass index, or BMI, compares your height and bone structure with your weight. If you are above or below your acceptable body mass then you should consider changing your diet and rate of activity.

Neither over-eating nor under-eating are good for your health as you get older. Try to be aware of your body's changing nutritional needs. Crash-dieting is not good for your long term health. If you have found yourself putting on weight in your thirties, forties and fifties you need to think about a change in lifestyle which includes food, drink and exercise. Excess weight is bad for your circulation and puts pressure on your vital organs. Enjoy your food and be active.

Otherwise you will look and feel miserable. And that is ageing in itself.

As with any diet advice if you have a personal history or family history of food intolerances, diabetes, high cholesterol levels or high blood pressure do seek advice from a health care professional to help you manage your diet safely.

Proteins

These are found in meat, fish, eggs, nuts, pulses and dairy products. They are essential for maintaining solid bones, building and maintaining muscle and for overall good health from the roots of your hair to the tips of your toenails. Early humans evolved from eating nuts and berries to become omnivorous diners who ate meat, fish and dairy produce too.

Some people find that they don't wish to eat heavy, meat-orientated meals as they get older or if their lifestyle becomes less active. Aim to eat small portions of good quality meat a few times a week, served with plenty of vegetables to add dietary fibre. Don't eat heavy, protein-rich meals just before bedtime. Allow your body time to digest your food.

A Mediterranean style diet which includes plenty of oily fish, such as mackerel, as well as fresh fish cooked on a barbecue or griddle, served with seasonal vegetables and salads, is also highly recommended. People living in Mediterranean countries such as Spain, Italy and Greece usually enjoy a diet that is rich in olive oil (see below). Some people believe this helps them to live longer and keep healthier.

Fats

It is very tempting in today's low fat world to believe that all fats are bad for you. How much total dietary fat does the average person need? To keep within safe limits you should:

- Consume less than 10% of your daily calories from saturated fats.

- Eat less than 300 mg of dietary cholesterol per day.

- Replace solid fats with oils, such as olive oil, when possible therefore reducing your calorie intake from solid fats.

Limit foods that contain synthetic sources of "trans fatty acids" such as hydrogenated oils and margarines, keeping your total trans fatty acid consumption as low as possible. After years of being warned of the cholesterol dangers of butter many of us now prefer it again- and we are right to do so – it is a natural food made from milk.

Olive oil is particularly characteristic of a Mediterranean diet. It contains a very high level of mono-unsaturated fats, most notably oleic acid, which medical studies suggest may be linked to a reduction in coronary heart disease risk. There is also evidence that the antioxidants in olive oil improve cholesterol regulation. Other benefits are anti-inflammatory and anti-hypertensive effects.

If this all sounds a bit technical then please use your common sense also. If you consume a fair amount of fatty food at breakfast or lunch then go easy for the rest of the day. That may mean cutting down on biscuits and cakes too, which often contain margarine or trans fatty acids. You can get round this by making your own teatime treats if you can't live without a bit of carbohydrate in your life!

Sugars and salts

Again the above are obviously to be found in cakes, puddings and biscuits. However these are also highly present in pre-packaged, made to be re-heated, supermarket ready meals. If they aren't it usually means that they have put in something even more despicable. If you don't believe me just try not eating these sorts of food for a few weeks and then buy a ready-made frozen lasagne or supermarket curry. All you will taste is sugar and salt. If you are keen to improve your eating habits but have a busy schedule think about cooking up a batch of your own ready meals and storing them in the freezer. You can then control the amount of sugar and salt in your meals.

Carbohydrates

Carbohydrates are found in bread, rice, pasta and potatoes in the form of sugars, starch and fibre; these foodstuffs are commonly used to bulk up meals and are often form a large proportion of the diets of rural or more peasant societies. Arguably in these societies the workers use more energy in manual labour and therefore are less likely to put on weight than those in sedentary "western" jobs and lifestyles.

The main function of carbohydrates is to provide our bodies with energy, especially the brain and the nervous system. An enzyme called amylase helps to turn carbohydrates into glucose (blood sugar), which is used for energy by the body. That is why we sometimes feel woozy and reach for the high energy snacks when we are hungry and our blood sugar is low. Beware of the quick hit effect of some carbohydrate rich snacks. Try eating some fruit as well and drinking plenty of water.

Some low carbohydrate diet plans suggest that one avoids "carbs" after 6 pm in the evening and more extreme weight loss diets eliminate them altogether for a period of time. If you subscribe to this kind of diet you may lose weight but you may also lack energy and lose your "mojo" as well. Instead try eating your main meal in the middle of the day (unfashionable in the UK and America, but the norm in France and the Mediterranean countries).

Dairy products

Most of us have known since childhood that milk is good for you. It contains calcium and protein to help build strong bones and teeth. With a choice of full fat, semi skimmed and skimmed milk now available there is no reason to leave milk out of your diet.

Depriving yourself of milk, cream and other dairy products because they might be "fattening" is not a good idea. If you feel that you should avoid cream cakes then try to eat good quality yoghurts instead. We still need calcium and protein as we get older to help maintain bone density and to avoid conditions such as osteoporosis which can leave post-menopausal or older women vulnerable to fractures.

Some people believe that they are allergic to milk and other dairy products; Sometimes this is in fact an intolerance of lactose, a sugar found in milk and other dairy products. Lactose intolerance can lead to bloating, discomfort and bowel problems. People with lactose intolerance do not have enough of the enzyme known as lactase to break down large quantities of lactose. Mammals other than humans lose the ability to process lactose after weaning. It is only certain human populations throughout the world that have developed the ability to process lactose into adulthood.

There are various non-invasive medical tests that can be used to diagnose genuine lactose intolerance. Dairies and supermarkets now offer a range of lactose free milk and dairy products. Allergy to the proteins found in milk is a different condition caused by an immune system reaction.

Fruit and vegetables

These are obviously very good for you and it's worth finding out how to maximize their potential. Many food experts suggest that eating fruit and vegetables that are in season gives the most benefits. For instance choose asparagus in the springtime and pumpkins in the autumn. Avoid buying over-packaged salad or vegetables that have been washed in strong chemicals and then sealed in cellophane.

If you can buy locally grown fruit and vegetables from a market stall or from a traditional greengrocer you should do so. Organically grown fruit and vegetables generally taste better and usually have a longer fridge or shelf life, as does the produce from allotments.

Try not to overcook vegetables, leave them a bit crunchy to benefit from the vitamins and minerals they contain. When you are cooking a stir-fry start with the really crunchy vegetables first, such as carrots, gradually adding onions, peppers, courgette, and mushrooms towards the end. Raw onion and garlic are also great immune system boosters.

Fruit and vegetables contain vitamin C which helps the absorption of iron; this is very important for women of all ages.

Some fruity tips

Apples are generally better crunched between meals or even at the beginning of a meal as the natural acidity of an apple can interfere with your digestion.

An orange a day keeps the doctor away. I like to halve, squeeze and drink the juice of at least one orange each morning to guarantee a burst of vitamin C. In fact I was advised to do this by a local lady during a particularly harsh winter in the French Alps when I mentioned a persistent sore throat and cough. It seems to work for me! I also find that commercial cartons of orange juice are often too tart; a real orange is much softer early in the morning.

Don't be tempted to drink too much concentrated fruit juice, especially without eating, as the acidity isn't great for your digestive juices or your teeth. Switch to water instead if you are avoiding alcohol or caffeine.

Vive la banane! Bananas make great snacks, they are sweet and filling. They also contain a good amount of potassium which always seems to settle the stomach after a little alcohol over-indulgence the night before! You can keep one in your handbag where it will ripen up nicely during the day.

Vegetarians and vegans

If you prefer a vegetarian or vegan diet (a vast percentage of the world's population is in fact vegetarian for economic or religious reasons) then do include nuts and pulses in your diet. Generally speaking vegetarians do not eat the flesh of mammals, birds or fish and they avoid animal fats too. Some vegetarians are quite happy to consume milk, eggs and cheese. Recent food scandals such as horsemeat in lasagnes, so-called "mad cow" disease and salmonella warnings connected with battery hen eggs have made many people more careful about what they eat.

Some people claim that a balanced vegetarian diet will help you look younger for longer as the body has to process fewer toxins. It is fair to say that many people who follow a vegetarian diet for health or ethical reasons often either abstain from or are moderate in their consumption of alcohol. Likewise they may be less likely to smoke, another activity that can cause premature ageing of the skin.

A person who follows a vegan diet does not eat the flesh of mammals, birds or fish, or any of their by-products which include animal fats, eggs, cheese and milk etc. If you decide to follow a vegan diet you need to ensure that your body is processing enough vitamins, especially A, B, B12, D as well as benefiting from calcium, iron and zinc. Many vegans take medically approved supplements to boost their immune system. Chick peas, lentils and kidney beans can all be combined with spices and vegetables to form the basis of tasty meat-free meals.

Keep hydrated

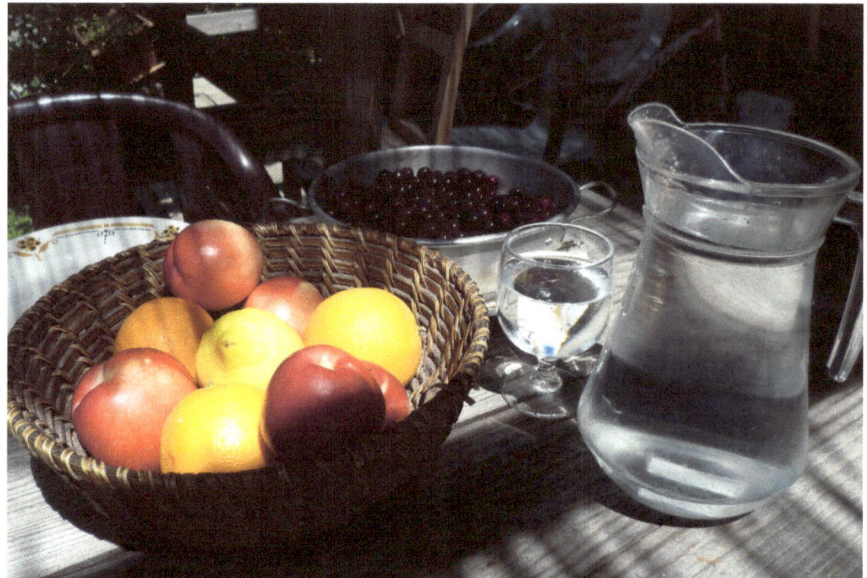

Drink at least two litres of water a day to keep your body hydrated

Many people just don't drink enough water. The average adult requires up to two litres of water per day. If you are exercising, working long hours or doing a job which requires a lot of talking you may need to drink even more. Dehydration actually causes part of the brain to shrink temporarily and interferes with some thought processes giving rise to headaches at the same time. Those headaches in turn make us frown, feel stressed and look stressed – very ageing.

Filtered or tap water is great, depending on the area you live in. Avoid buying or keeping water in plastic bottles. As the plastic bottle heats up or cools down, especially if you are carrying water in your car, dangerous chemical changes occur in the composition of the plastic which many people now believe can cause cancer related problems. Try to carry your drinking water in a thermos style flask which you can wash out thoroughly after each use.

Don't fool yourself with sparkling waters, fruit juices, tea or coffee (nice treats as they are). Tea and coffee have diuretic qualities – that is they encourage the excretion of water from the body, making you want to go to the toilet more often, therefore having a dehydrating effect. If you can't resist these treats then remember to drink a glass of water on the side. This is often a good idea if you are drinking alcohol too. Just have a glass of ordinary still water (tap or glass bottle) for every few glasses of wine!

Exercise helps

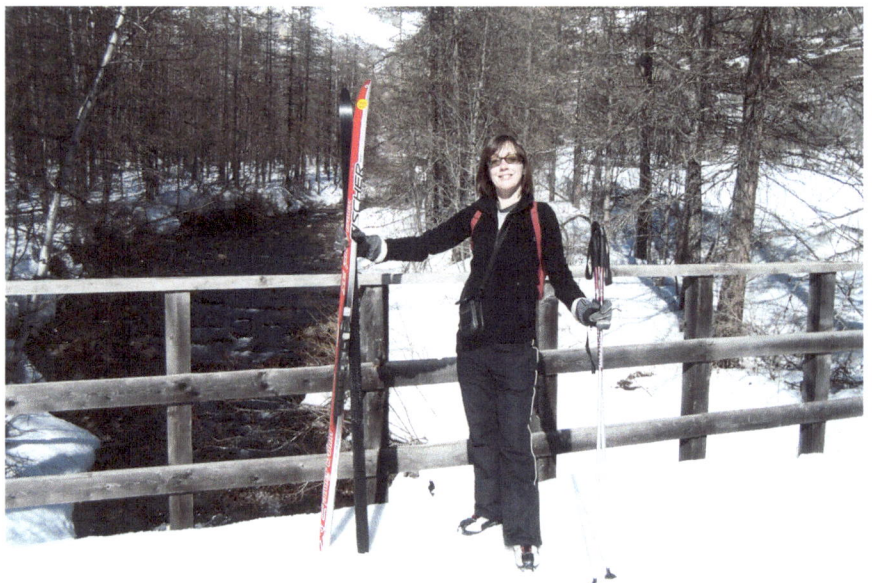

Cross country skiing – energetic exercise in the fresh air

Regular exercise is the best way to feel good and look younger. Exercise helps the blood to circulate around the body, making the heart and lungs work better. Regular exercise also helps to maintain strong bones and joints and to build muscle to support them. A good regime can protect against the ageing effects of arthritis, rheumatism and osteoporosis.

Homo sapiens was intended by nature to be a hunter-gatherer. Our bodies are designed to move, run and throw things. However in the world of office work and the Internet, many of us are less active than ever.

Exercise for your body shape

As we discussed in the chapter about body shape, different types of exercise with different ultimate goals can be adapted to suit tall thin people (ectomorphs), muscular, athletic types (mesomorphs) and shorter, stockier people (endomorphs).

Long, tall ectomorphs find it quite difficult to put on muscle or fat. Ectomorph ladies may bemoan their lack of cleavage but we are all envious of their long legs and slim, toned arms. Ectomorphs need to eat regularly and keep up their calorie intake. They may enjoy swimming or cycling, circuit or even light weight training as a means to bulk up a bit.

Athletic mesomorphs sometimes find that exercise makes them bulk up too much, and a high calorie intake can lead them to putting on weight. Mesomorphs need to exercise in proportion to their calorie intake.

Endomorphs don't build muscle easily but they can tone up with walking, cycling, gentle aerobics, swimming, tennis, yoga etc.

Indoors and outdoors

If you live in a town or city going to the gym or the swimming pool may be the easiest way to keep fit. Some people are motivated by exercising with other people, others prefer a solitary run or cycle ride. Choose a form of exercise that suits your needs and your schedule. There are many devices available on the market that measure how far you've walked, run or cycled if you need that incentive.

Country dwellers are luckier than town dwellers in many ways, but wherever you live being active is an essential part of keeping healthy and looking good. Owning a dog or walking dogs for other people is a great way of getting some exercise and gives you that incentive to get out of the house. You can vary your exercise according to the season. Alpine (downhill) skiing and cross country skiing are fabulous ways of enjoying the winter sunshine and the mountains. If you think that skiing is a little extreme for you why not try snowshoeing in the valleys instead?

Getting started

If you are just starting to exercise after a period of not exercising much because of illness or pregnancy, take it easy at first, build up a regular programme gently and do have some rest days. It is important to listen to your body. If you are really out of condition visit your GP before you start exercising to have your heart monitored and your blood pressure checked.

Some helpful hints:

On days that I work from home I sometimes choose a quick morning run for my exercise if I'm short of time, or a longer more leisurely afternoon walk if I've accomplished all my tasks in the morning.

On days that I've worked away from home a quick run in the early evening is very refreshing. I currently live at quite a high altitude (1200 metres above sea-level) so warming up and cooling down is an important part of my routine. It 's very easy to become breathless so I often mix my running and walking as I warm up i.e. walk 30 paces, run 30 paces, walk 40 paces, run 40 paces.

Beware of over-exercising if you want to avoid your body looking too taut and muscular. A gaunt, hollow-cheeked look because you have denied your body food and adequate rest is probably not what you are aiming for.

Yoga and Pilates

Both of these disciplines will help you to attain good posture and core strength. (Your core is the trunk of your body; the chest, stomach, hips and back). If you practise yoga or Pilates regularly you will exercise all your muscle groups and will feel stronger when you are taking part in sporting activities such as running, swimming, skiing, tennis etc.

Yoga is a fantastic discipline because a good yoga teacher will explain to you about the breathing required to help oxygenate the muscles and the body during the exercises. For those who tend to suffer from stress it is true that yoga has a very calming effect, which in itself is anti-ageing. (Please refer also to the section below about Sleep and Relaxation).

Sleep and relaxation

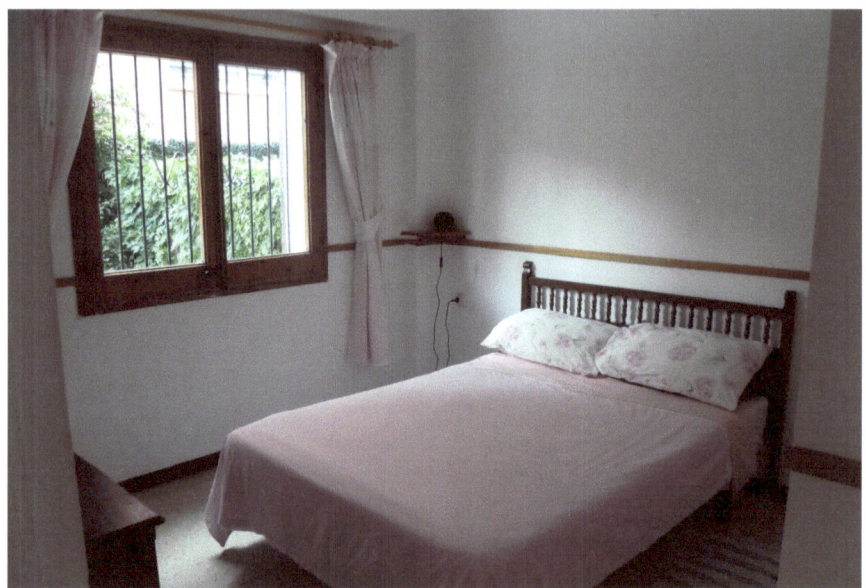

Create a calm ambiance in your bedroom – no televisions or laptops please!

Don't under-estimate the importance of sleep and relaxation in staying young and looking young. Try to get at least 8 hours sleep a night; 10 hours is even better. Your body needs this time asleep to repair itself and so does your brain.

How we all marvelled in the 1980s at Margaret Thatcher, the Iron Lady and the UK's first female prime minister when she said she only needed a few hours sleep every night. I have worked with people who did likewise and noticed that eventually lack of sleep caused illness, immune system problems and in some cases depression or dependence on stimulants.

Those of us who have survived the sleep deprivation caused by babies and small children will be grateful for moving on from that phase. The constant jet-lag feeling of only getting a few hours sleep here or there is never pleasant. Although dealing with the strange time schedules and needs of teenagers can be equally challenging.

The different stages of sleep

Human sleep is divided into two types: rapid eye movement (REM) and non-rapid eye movement (NREM or non-REM) sleep. The American Academy of Sleep Medicine further divides NREM into three stages: N1, N2, and N3.

NREM stage 1: This is a stage between sleep and wakefulness. Muscles are active, and the eyes roll slowly, opening and closing moderately.

NREM stage 2: In this stage it gradually becomes harder to awaken the sleeper; the alpha waves of the previous stage are interrupted by abrupt activity called sleep spindles and K-complexes.

NREM stage 3: This stage is called slow-wave sleep (SWS). The sleeper is less responsive to the environment; many environmental stimuli produce no reactions.

REM: The sleeper now enters the rapid eye movement phase where most muscles are paralyzed. REM sleep is activated by acetylcholine secretion and is inhibited by neurons that secrete serotonin. Oxygen consumption by the brain is higher than when the sleeper is awake. An adult reaches REM approximately every 90 minutes, with the latter half of sleep being more dominated by this stage. The function of REM sleep is uncertain but a lack of it will impair the ability to learn complex tasks.

Sleep continues in cycles of REM and NREM, usually four or five of them per night, the order normally being N1 → N2 → N3 → N2 → REM. There is a greater amount of deep sleep (stage N3) earlier in the night, while the proportion of REM sleep increases in the two cycles just before natural awakening.

Avoiding sleep problems

Insomnia can be a problem as we get older and have more responsibilities. Sometimes it is very difficult to switch off from the events of the day, financial worries, things you have to do tomorrow etc. Many of us live more and more in a non-stop 24 hour world. Some people have to work night shifts or irregular hours.

Here are some sensible suggestions for a good night's sleep:

Try to make it a golden rule not to take your phone or laptop to bed. Do not work beyond what you deem to be a reasonable time, depending on your schedule.

Make a list of the things you need to do tomorrow so that you feel organised and put it to one side until the morning. Most tasks are tackled much better after a good night's sleep.

Do your best to unwind for at least 30 minutes before you go to bed, choose a book, magazine or TV program that is "light", perhaps with humorous or undemanding subject matter.

Do not eat a heavy meal just before bedtime and avoid caffeinated drinks such as tea and coffee in the evening.

Make sure you have taken some exercise and fresh air earlier in the day.

A warm bath with appropriately scented candles can help put you in the mood for sleep.

Spend some time actually talking with your partner if you are in a relationship! Making love is a good way to release sleep-inducing endorphins too.

Relaxation and dealing with stress

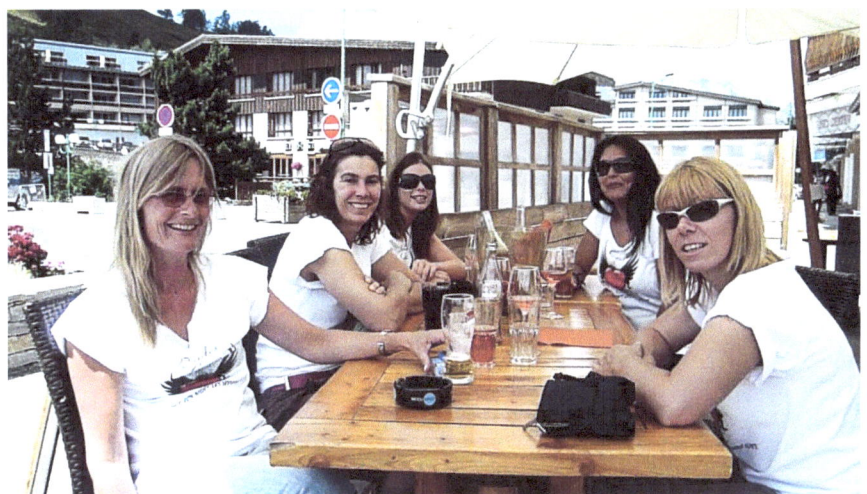

Friends and laughter – a great tonic

Even if you have a very busy life do try to find some time each week for sport or feel-good activities such as singing, dancing or art. Different people have different ways of unwinding. Have you ever noticed how a lot of creative people seem to stay younger looking than their contemporaries? Another tried and tested way of relaxing is to meet up with your female friends for drinks, food and a jolly good giggle. Laughter releases those feel-good endorphins and makes you feel good about yourself. If there's dancing later, all the better!

Funnily enough we all need a little stress in our lives. It is part of what makes us get up off our backsides to work and achieve our goals. If family life can seem stressful it is only because most of us care about doing the best for our loved ones. It is how we deal with stress and turn it to our advantage that is important.

Making lists to help you prioritize is essential. The people who are most successful in their work and everyday lives plan ahead, therefore avoiding stressful clashes of commitments. Use a diary, filofax or software program to plan out your weeks, days and daily appointments. Shopping lists are life-savers too; keep a piece of paper or a whiteboard in your kitchen so you can write down items that you need to buy.

Many people who want to live calmer lives enjoy learning relaxation techniques such as yoga and meditation. Yoga originated in ancient India and became popular in the western world (Europe, USA and Australasia) from the 1960s onwards. You do not have to subscribe to any particular religious faith to practise yoga. The physical exercises are combined with beneficial breathing exercises to contribute to mental calmness and alertness. Yoga teachers usually belong to an organisation called The Wheel of Yoga. It is worth trying out a few different classes near to where you live to choose one that suits you.

Meditation exists in many forms. It forms the basis of spiritual contemplation in many of the world's leading religions such as Christianity, Hinduism and Buddhism. However you do not have to be religious to practise meditation.

During the late 1960s and 1970s transcendental meditation (TM) became popular in western civilizations. Like yoga, TM takes its origins from the practices of holy men in India but it has been adapted to suit all nationalities and lifestyles. TM combines breath control and a personal mantra given by a trained TM teacher. People who practise TM regularly say that it puts their body and mind into a calm state, while still being aware of their surroundings. They feel more focused and refreshed after meditation. Some people also claim (with good evidence) that transcendental meditation keeps them looking and feeling younger.

Your skin

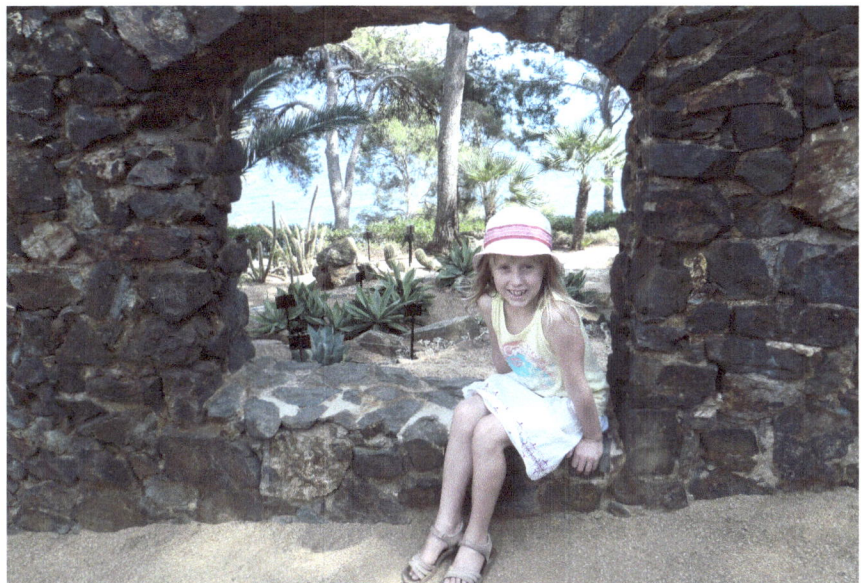

It's never too early to learn about protecting your skin from the sun

Your skin reflects the overall health of your body. Most of us start life with lovely moist plump, quite unblemished skin. As we age our skin becomes less elastic due to hormonal changes and the loss of collagen, the protein found in connective tissue.

Sometimes the weight gain and subsequent weight loss of pregnancy can leave us with skin that is less elastic than before. Most women find that by their forties or fifties their skin seems thinner and less "plump" than before. Lines appear and jaw-lines sag a little.

A balanced diet with sufficient protein, dairy products or equivalents and fresh vegetables can help you maintain a good healthy weight in proportion to your height and bone structure. Your skin will also look better if you have fairly firm, toned muscles beneath it, so gentle exercise is important. Remember that drastic weight loss diets do not help your health or skin. It is also very important to keep your body hydrated by drinking plenty of water throughout the day.

Moisturise, moisturise, moisturise...

A light moisturiser applied in the morning and a richer cream at night will do wonders for your skin. Some of the classic (and not too expensive) brands such as Ponds or Olay are completely sufficient for most women. If you live in a dry climate or spend many hours in centrally heated or air conditioned buildings this is very important. If you live in a more humid climate or near the sea, you may find that your skin is naturally quite moist and you can use less moisturiser.

Anti-ageing creams

Very few rigorous scientific surveys have been carried out on these products. Most manufacturers and advertisers use the phrase "can reduce the appearance of fine lines and wrinkles" when marketing their products. There has been a lot of interest lately in creams that stimulate the production of collagen. In 2013 it was claimed that creams containing peptides or protein fragments such as Matrixyl could improve the firmness and plumpness of skin by penetrating the skin's outer layer and stimulating collagen production.

A clinical trial in 2012 found that in a sample group of people, aged 45-80 years old, nearly half of those who used Boots No.7 Protect and Perfect with peptides for six months reported a visible improvement in skin elasticity and firmness compared with 22% of the people using an "ordinary" moisturiser. Draw your own conclusions from this. Maybe there are simply benefits from a regular skin care regime and facial massage? If you are curious to try anti-ageing collagen stimulating creams for yourself, popular products are currently the Olay Regenerist range or the St.Ives Collagen Elastin Facial Moisturiser as well as Boots No.7 Protect and Perfect. I offer no guarantees however!

Skincare experts still emphasise that avoiding over exposure to the sun and not smoking are the most effective ways to keep your skin looking young.

Let your skin breathe sometimes

Some women feel that they have to wear the complete moisturiser, foundation and blusher combination to be fully dressed. Unfortunately some jobs, such as hospitality work, air stewardess or actress, pretty much demand a full face of slap! Do let your skin breathe in between assignments and try to find really light easy-to-wear products.

Even if it is just a walk to the corner shop do try to get out into the fresh air, it is the best tonic for your complexion. Use your weekends and time off to get out into the countryside if you live in the town during the rest of the week. Walking, cycling, jogging – these are all activities which will put some colour in your cheeks and help your complexion.

Exposure to the sun

My friends and I were talking recently about how naive we were about sunbathing back in the 1970s and 1980s. Moderate sun exposure in a mild climate helps our bodies to make and store vitamin D. Prolonged exposure to intense sun, resulting in sunburn, is not good for us.

You need to be aware of your skin type. People with black, Asian or Mediterranean skin are usually more able to cope with sustained exposure to the sun. These ethnic groups have more melanin in their skin than others. Many people believe that the olive oil and fruit in a traditional Mediterranean diet also helps to condition the skin, keep it moist and promote a healthy tan. Paler, dryer northern European skins are prone to redness and burning in a relatively short time.

Allowing your skin to burn can lead to problems in the future, such as skin cancer, due to long-term skin damage. Beware of thinking that just because you have smothered yourself in factor 30 or 50 sun cream you can stay out in the sun all day and that you are safe from all those harmful ultraviolet rays. Sun creams make you feel that you can stand more sun on your skin but many experts now believe that the chemicals in sun creams could be harmful too.

There are two main types of damaging ultraviolet sunlight: UVA and UVB. UVB rays are absorbed by the top layer of skin or epidermis. This causes sun tanning but also burning. UVA rays penetrate deeper into the skin, damaging the middle layer or dermis. The dermis contains the elastic tissues that keep the skin stretchy. UVA rays therefore have the effect of ageing the skin and causing wrinkles on the face and the body.

The delicate skin of our décolletage (chest and breasts) is particularly vulnerable to the sun. Some older women who have been sun worshippers in the past are left with blotchy, uneven, wrinkled skin on their bosom with burst blood vessels near the surface. This damage cannot be fully repaired by surgery. The best improvement that specialist skin surgeons can achieve is by using laser treatments to burn off the top layer of damaged skin. They will also try to stimulate new cell growth in the dermis. These "resurfacing" treatments are expensive, easily costing thousands of pounds or dollars and are also time consuming.

People with this much skin damage will be warned by their surgeon and other skin care professionals to keep out of the sun for the rest of their lives and to keep covered up. This is a huge price to pay for being blasé about sun tanning in your youth.

Another part, or rather parts, of your body where the skin shows its age very quickly are your hands. If you think about it your hands are always exposed to the sun in summer and the cold in winter. The skin becomes quite thin, even in our twenties, and also gets dried out easily. Always apply plenty of suntan lotion to the top of your hands to prevent deep lines, wrinkles and brown spots (commonly known as liver spots) when out and about in the summer or on holiday. I bet Joan Collins wears smart white gloves when she goes to the beach nowadays. Apply hand cream after doing household tasks such as washing up and wear rubber gloves if necessary. Be particularly zealous in the winter months.

In truth if you have pale skin, and want to tan safely, very gradual exposure of well moisturised skin to the sunshine is the best way forward. Be prepared to cover up and find some shade before your skin starts to feel too warm. This is common sense. A good rule for everyone is to always have a hat with a brim to hand to avoid sunstroke. Protect the delicate skin around your eyes by wearing the more "wraparound" style of sunglasses with good quality UV filter lenses. Use a moisturiser with a suitable level of sun protection for your skin type even on cloudier days.

Smoking is not good for your skin (or your health)

Why spend loads of money on clothes, haircuts and make-up if you are going to walk around smelling like an ashtray and looking older than your biological age?

Slightly harsh I know but smoking causes premature ageing of the skin and the best way to combat this is to give up the habit! Moreover smoking can cause lung cancer and heart disease. Cigarette smoke contains over 4000 toxins, many of which are absorbed directly into the bloodstream and are carried into the skin's structure by the blood. Smoking also makes the blood vessels in the top layers of the skin constrict, reducing the oxygen levels in the blood. This also reduces the levels of collagen in the skin giving rise to deep wrinkles around the eyes, mouth and neck.

If you are a confirmed smoker do try to cut down or alternatively try using one of the electronic cigarettes or nicotine vaporisers which bypass the need for tobacco. Or just give up altogether! More and more of my female friends have given up smoking in the last few years. If you can't or don't want to give up, it's your life and ultimately your choice, just don't be ignorant of the facts.

Your teeth

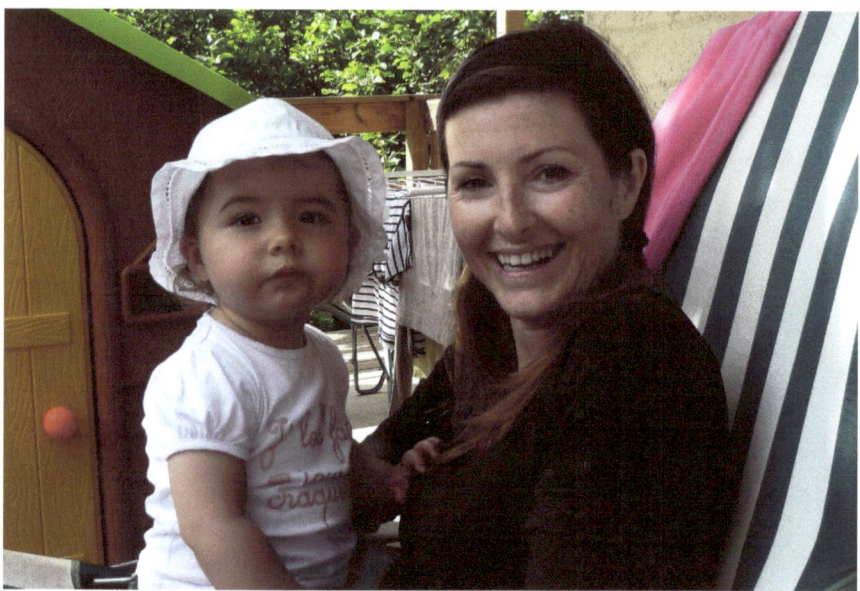

Not a model – a 44 year old woman with well-maintained teeth and a great smile

There is nothing more ageing than bad teeth or missing teeth. If you are going to have good teeth in middle and older age you need to start looking after your teeth and gums from childhood. Having grown up in the 1970s with parents who put a lot of cakes on the table, added sugar to cereals and in cups of tea I had far too many fillings by the time I was in my early twenties. I had to unlearn a few bad habits and take more care of my teeth as an adult. If you are already the mother or grandmother of young children take note and help them to look after their teeth from the start.

Anyway, back to us ladies who want to stay looking young! If you want to have strong teeth eat a good healthy diet with sufficient protein and calcium. Avoid too much sugar, carbohydrates and those ever so tempting energy drinks. Natural fruit juices are very acidic and dentists now say that drinking too much juice can weaken the enamel (outer layer) of our teeth. Smoking and excessive alcohol are also bad for your teeth. Heavy smokers often end up with stained yellowy brown teeth due to the nicotine in cigarettes. Tea and coffee unfortunately also stain the teeth.

Brushing and flossing

Clean your teeth twice a day, in the morning and evening. A tip: I sometimes carry a little travelling toothbrush with me if I'm out and about during the day. If I'm having lunch with friends and going on somewhere afterwards I don't like to find bits of my lunch between my teeth at afternoon tea time! Sugar-free chewing gum is a handy alternative for making your teeth feel clean and your breath nice and fresh after a meal.

Brush your top teeth from the upper gum downwards and your lower teeth from the lower gum upwards. Never brush the gum away from the teeth. Make sure you clean behind your teeth as this is where calcium deposits known as plaque build up, making it difficult to clean the tooth and gum adequately. Don't just pay attention to the front teeth; make sure you clean the molars and pre-molars towards the back of your mouth. Use a toothbrush with a smaller head to get into difficult areas. Whether you use a traditional or electric toothbrush is a matter of personal taste. Bleeding gums are a sign that you should see your dentist. They have also been linked to a higher risk of heart disease.

Flossing is a really good way to get to those awkward little spaces between your teeth where food collects and decays! I wish I had known about flossing when I was a teenager. If you don't have perfectly spaced "Hollywood" teeth you may find that either the satin tape floss or the more traditional stringy floss really helps. I tend to floss once a day in the evening after brushing my teeth and then finish off with a rinse of mouthwash, then water. Some people floss more often, for others once every few days is sufficient. It is normal to see a little blood if you floss your teeth.

Dental treatments

Opinions are divided about whitening toothpastes that you can buy at chemists or supermarkets. Some dentists claim that the active ingredients have a detrimental long term effect on the enamel of the teeth with little actual improvement to the appearance of the teeth. Whitening treatments undertaken at a dentist's surgery can be a good idea if you are planning a special occasion such as a wedding or have work events where you want to look your absolute best.

Current health guidelines suggest that we visit the dentist twice a year for a check up and to have our teeth professionally cleaned by a hygienist if necessary. Many dentists nowadays work in conjunction with a hygienist as this gives them more time to concentrate on the medical side of dentistry, fillings, crowns etc.

If you have neglected your teeth for a number of years and they are in a very bad state or perhaps an accident has damaged your teeth and gums, you may consider having some or all of your unhealthy teeth removed and replacing them with screw-in tooth implants. This requires a certain level of commitment; there is surgery under a full anaesthetic, it is expensive and painful during the recovery time. Many people however are pleased with the results and prefer this to wearing conventional dentures or false teeth.

As in all things health and beauty orientated do remember that "prevention is better than a cure."

Your eyes

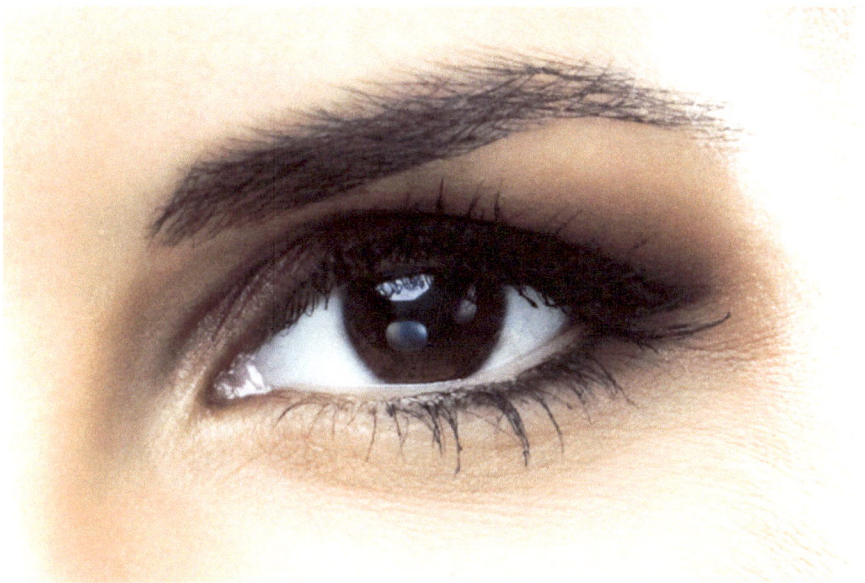

Clear, sparkling eyes are the result of a healthy lifestyle

Some lucky people enjoy perfect vision for many years while others have to deal with being near-sighted or far-sighted from childhood. However many people find that as they approach forty their eyesight changes and that they need to use reading glasses for the first time. Don't be daunted by the idea of having to wear glasses or contact lenses as you get older. It's really not the end of the world!

Far-sightedness (hyperopia)

People who are far-sighted see things at a distance more easily than they see things up close. Far-sightedness occurs when light entering the eye is focused behind the retina instead of directly on it. This is because the eye is too short or the cornea is not curved enough, or the lens sits farther back in the eye than normal. Younger people with a tendency towards far-sightedness often don't need glasses or contact lenses as the lens of the eye, which is flexible, automatically becomes rounder to bring near objects into focus or more flat to bring distant objects into focus.

As we approach our forties the lens of the eye loses some of its flexibility (this is called presbyopia). At this point glasses or contact lenses become necessary.

Near-sightedness (myopia)

Near-sighted or short-sighted people can see objects that are very close up but have difficulty focusing on objects in the distance. Most near-sightedness is caused by a natural change in the shape of the eyeball. Sometimes it can be caused by a change in the cornea or the lens. These characteristics cause light rays entering the eye to focus in front of the retina rather than on the retina itself. Glasses or contact lenses are used to correct the problem. Some people opt for laser eye surgery for a more permanent correction, but this is not suitable for everyone. It works best for people who have recorded only slight changes in their eyesight from year to year.

How to keep your eyes healthy

Consult an optician or ophthalmologist if you notice changes in your vision. If you do need to wear glasses or contact lenses make sure you have a full eye test carried out by a qualified ophthalmologist. They will also examine your eyes for any signs of cataracts (cloudy areas on the lens of the eye) or glaucoma (eye diseases which damage the optic nerve). If you already wear glasses or contact lenses make sure your prescription is up-to-date. Have a check up at least every two years.

If you have been short-sighted most of your life (like me!) you may find that as you reach your forties you become less able to read small print close up. It's not that you're becoming far-sighted it is simply the lens of the eye becoming less flexible. Bifocal or varifocal glasses are very useful at this point; these have a distance prescription at the top and centre of the lens and the reading prescription towards the bottom. You can now also buy varifocal and bifocal disposable contact lenses, although they are fairly expensive.

You can adapt your diet to include nutrients such as omega-3 fatty acids, lutein, zinc, and vitamins C and E which may prevent age-related vision problems such as macular degeneration and cataracts. Helpful foods are: green, leafy vegetables such as spinach and kale; salmon, tuna and other oily fish; eggs, nuts, beans and other non-meat protein sources; citrus fruits, such as oranges and fruit juices. You should stop smoking as soon as possible if you want to look after your eyes. Smoking makes you more likely to suffer from cataracts, optic nerve damage, and macular degeneration.

It's a good idea to wear sunglasses outdoors to avoid too much exposure to UV rays which can cause cataracts and macular degeneration. Choose sunglasses that block 99% - 100% of both UVA and UVB rays. Wraparound lenses help to protect your eyes from the side. Polarized lenses reduce glare when you are driving. Some contact lenses offer UV protection however it's advisable to wear sunglasses for extra protection, especially in bright sunlight.

Always use safety eyewear at home or work if using hazardous materials. Wear eye protection while playing hardball sports such as hockey and choose good quality goggles for winter sports. Don't stare at computer screens for too long or you could experience eyestrain, blurry vision, dry eyes as well as headaches, neck, shoulder or back pain.

Nowadays it is easy to choose glasses that suit your face, lifestyle and budget. In my experience you do get what you pay for in terms of the durability of frames. Some high street opticians offer a two for one deal so that you can select one style for everyday wear and perhaps a more fun style for evening wear. If you have quite delicate features there are some very lightweight glasses available with almost invisible frames. However some women like the dark-framed "sexy librarian" look and boldly wear their glasses as a fashion accessory.

Your hair

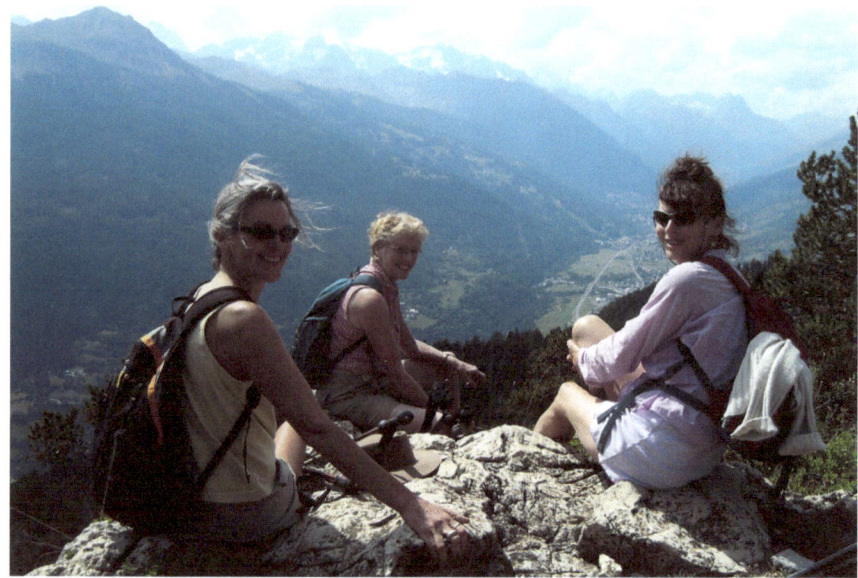

Ladies in their forties and fifties – different hair colours, different styles

Several factors determine the behaviour of your hair as you get older. First of all there is your genetic inheritance i.e. type of hair, whether it is fine, coarse, curly etc. Often genetic inheritance dictates whether you will start to see white hairs in your twenties, thirties or much later on. Life-style factors such as smoking, excessive drinking, stress and poor diet can make hair brittle and damaged. Over-frequent perming, straightening or colouring of your hair causes it to dry out leading to split ends and frizz.

To dye or not to dye?

It's a fact that some women look fabulous in their sixties and seventies with naturally white or grey hair. (Think Honor Blackman, Helen Mirren and Judi Dench).

Nature is a little tough on brunettes and ladies with black hair as those first white hairs, caused by a simple change in levels of pigmentation as we age, start showing much earlier. But you can have fun trying out a variety of hair colours, from chestnut to more burgundy shades, either administered at home or at the salon. If you want a natural look do stay as close to your original hair colour as possible, as this will always be a better match for your skin. Use temporary wash-in wash-out hair colour to try out new looks. Many products nowadays use less ammonia and are more oil-based.

Owners of blonde or so-called mousy hair, which often has a multitude of different colours and tones, can make use of subtle highlights and lowlights in their hair during their forties and fifties. As your hair gains more of a percentage of white, you can tweak the additional colours to keep your hair more golden blonde or light brown.

You can't have long hair after 40...

Utter rubbish! If you want to wear your hair long and it grows easily and it suits your look and lifestyle... go for it!

It is fair to say, however, that the naturally long unkempt hair or the extreme styles that some of us sported in our youth are less flattering when we get older as our faces change shape and our skin loses its elasticity. A friend of mine in her fifties, who has always worn her blonde hair long with a centre parting, now asks her hairdresser to cut a few shorter jaw-level lengths at the front to soften her style when she ties her hair back. This is very subtle and flattering and gives a much more youthful appearance.

If you have naturally fine hair you should aim for regular haircuts (every six to eight weeks), whatever its length, in order to eliminate wispy ends and to add volume. A jaw or shoulder length bob is often easy to manage and ideal for the professional woman or the busy mum who has children /work/ elderly parents to organise and not much time for herself.

Hair changes in pregnancy or due to illness

Pregnancy hormones make a woman's hair appear thicker while she is "expecting" but the downside is sometimes quite radical hair loss during the first few months of your baby's life. If this happens to you don't feel downhearted just go to your hairdresser and have a shorter cut, with a few layers put in until your hair regains its normal state – and it always does.

Understandably a major fear of many people undergoing treatment for cancer is the hair loss associated with chemotherapy. Many women choose to crop their hair or shave their head at the first sign of hair loss, often with considerable support from their family and friends. Some people opt for wearing a wig or headscarf during the treatment period, others just "go commando" when and where they feel comfortable.

You will now find numerous videos on YouTube and other Internet platforms documenting hair loss and re-growth during cancer treatment. Generally speaking some baby soft hair starts to grow back about 16 weeks after the end of chemotherapy. Some people do experience a change in hair texture after treatment of this kind, and adapt their new hairstyle accordingly.

Make-up and grooming

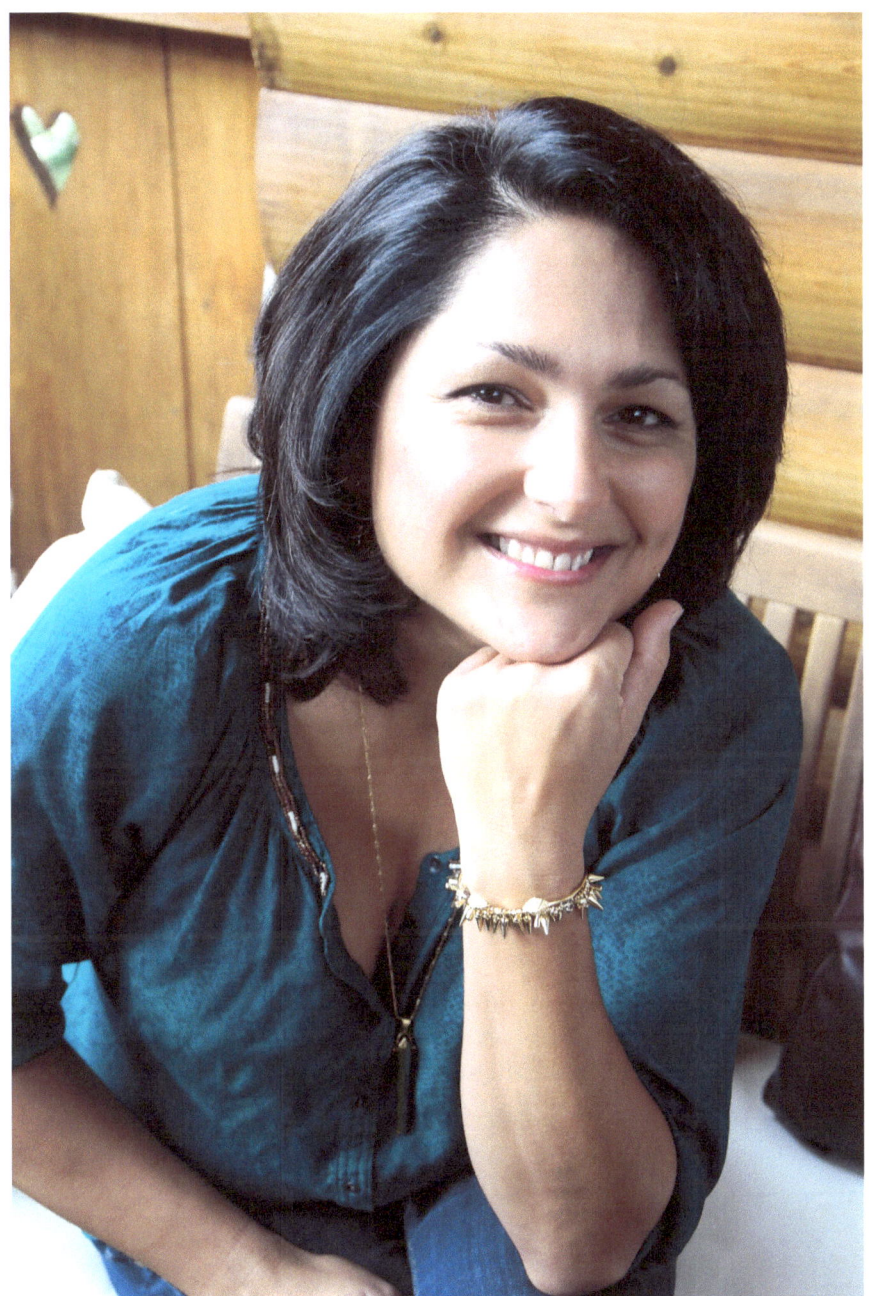

Feeling confident in your forties, with glowing skin and subtle make-up

In our teenage years we probably experimented with all sorts of different looks: disco, hippy, punk, gothic, New Romantic, grunge, 1950s etc, depending on our fashion and musical tastes. A few remarkable people such as Vivienne Westwood and Zandra Rhodes continue to wear quite outrageous make-up well into their sixties and seventies. For most of us once we reach our late twenties and thirties we have a make-up routine organised which suits our adult personality and lifestyle.

The key to looking after your skin as you get older is, as we have already discussed, avoiding too much sunshine, being a non-smoker and using a good moisturiser regularly. As we get older the idea of "less is more" comes into play. Some skin care experts suggest that we should avoid heavier, cream-based make up as we get older because it tends to emphasise the wrinkles in mature skins, especially around the eyes and mouth. They favour a good moisturiser and a light powder foundation.

It's always worth booking an appointment with a make-up specialist who has experience of working with mature complexions. They will be able to demonstrate the latest foundations, blushers, eye-shadows and lip colours which will suit your skin type and colouring.

As we get older we may find that our lips are less plump than when we were younger. We may want to tone down the scarlet reds that we wore in our thirties, which complemented our youthful complexions and hairstyles, to a more subtle orangey red, pinky red or burnt red to give a softer, more flattering lip colour.

Glossy colours reflect more light and can make the lips look plumper, giving a more youthful impression. Defining the outside of the lips just beyond their natural line with a lip pencil and then filling in with a lipstick of a very similar colour is another useful trick.

Beware of over-plucking your eyebrows as you get older, as the effect can be ageing. The trend these days is for quite dark, natural looking eyebrows. Use an eyebrow pencil in a shade which suits your natural hair colour to create thicker eyebrows if yours have become a bit sparse.

If you have particular colours of eye-shadow that you like consider whether the tone and the finish (pearly, matt or glittery) still suits you as you get older. Blue eye-shadow against blue eyes can be too overpowering; try nude shades and browns instead to enhance your eyes rather than overwhelming them. For brown or green eyes, subtle shades of light blue can really liven up the eye area. Lilacs and mauves can be an interesting colour choice, but avoid these if you have large or rather puffy eyelids as it can look as if your eyes are simply tired or red. Choose your eye-shadow to complement your eye colour, skin tone and hair, rather than matching it to your outfit.

False eyelashes are great fun for a really special night out but I don't think many of us more mature ladies will be wearing them to the supermarket like the young Essex girls do. Beware of overdoing kohl and mascara as you get older. Perhaps change from absolute black to brown/black for a more subtle effect. However "beauty is in the eye of the beholder" and if you are an attention seeking make-up wearer by nature, and can handle the attention, why stop because you've reached a certain age?

Edit your wardrobe

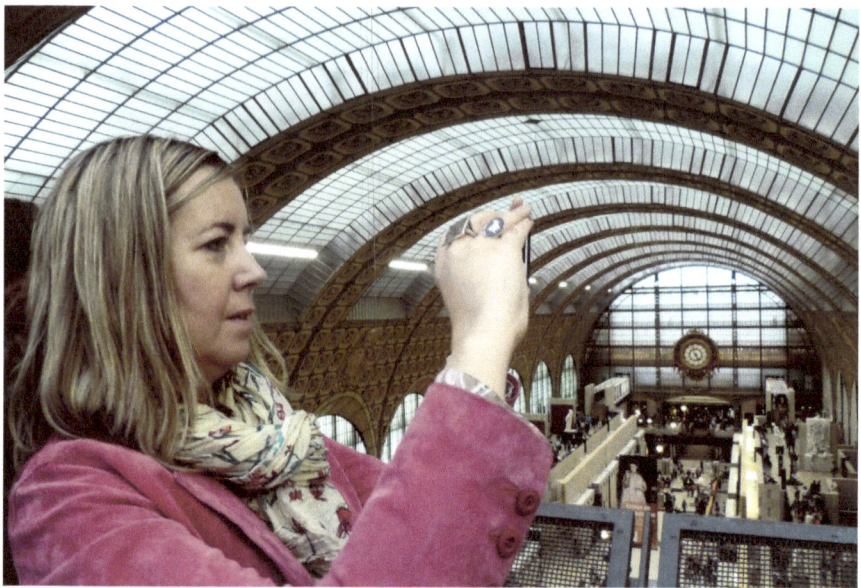

Looking chic in the city, with a flattering pink jacket and a pretty scarf

What you wear and what you have in your wardrobe will depend on your current job, your lifestyle and where you live. You can still wear fashionable, well cut clothes in your forties, fifties, sixties, seventies and beyond.

I'm not a great fan of makeover shows which remove every pair of jeans and handy, practical fleeces from a woman's wardrobe. How do you walk your dog in stilettos and a lovely structured jacket/ dress combination? Unless you're a chic Parisienne with a dog that lives in your handbag of course, in which case you won't need my lifestyle advice anyway!

So if you want to preserve the aura of youthfulness here are a few ideas to consider:

Don't wear clothes that are too tight; be prepared to buy a size larger if you like a particular "youthful" trend. You will feel more comfortable too.

Pick out styles that you like in fashion magazines or browse around the "younger" high street shops and then look for similar items in the more "age appropriate" shops. It's handy if you've got a teenage daughter or younger friend to go shopping with too.

Do get yourself properly measured and fitted for bras to suit your figure and lifestyle. Some women also swear by undergarments with bit of spandex to give themselves a flatter stomach and smaller waist.

Dress to suit your character. Joan Collins is fabulous at being Joan Collins, some of us may be able to carry off her international well-dressed actress style, others will be happy just dressing up a simple outfit with a scarf or a nice jacket when appropriate. If you've always been a rock chick why stop now? There's nothing wrong with sporting a rock star T-shirt teamed with a smart pair of black jeans, great jewellery, heels and artfully tousled hair.

As you get older think carefully about the colour and tone of the clothes you wear, especially the colours that you put close to your face. Your hair and skin tone will probably change from your thirties onwards. Black is always chic, but can be draining for the complexion as you get older, so team a black top with a bright scarf at the neck or choose a sophisticated black and white design instead.

You don't have to opt for beige and neutrals just because you have reached a certain age. The current trend for neon colours brings zest to a more mature complexion and looks great with all hair colours including grey or white. I bought a simple neon pink/orange vest top this summer and wore it with cropped jeans on many occasions. It was such a "feel-good" item of clothing; complete strangers used to smile at me when I walked into shops and cafés. If you are red-headed you may want to avoid a colour clash between your crowning glory and a neon pink T-shirt by opting for lemon or lime instead. Although there are wonderful exceptions to every rule!

Try to accentuate the parts of your body you feel most comfortable with. Again, exercise, fresh air and a light tan or healthy colour will give you more confidence to work those outfits you've put together. Finally do remember: you're never fully dressed without a smile!

The menopause – a new beginning?

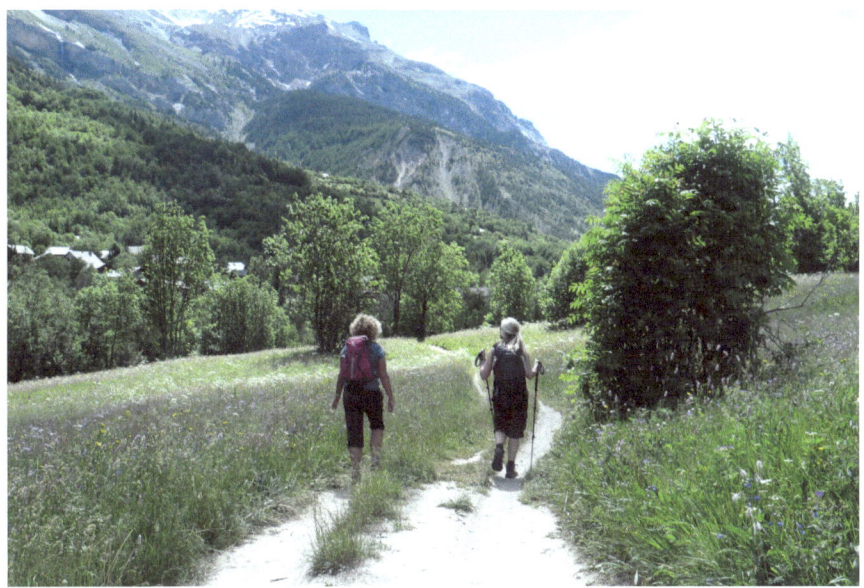

Regular exercise during the menopause years helps to maintain healthy bones and muscles

Most women experience the menopause during their late 40s or early 50s, and it indicates the end of the fertile phase of a woman's life. The menopause is most accurately defined as the permanent cessation of the primary functions of the ovaries. These are the ripening and release of eggs (ova) and the release of hormones that bring about the creation of the uterine lining, plus the subsequent shedding of the uterine lining which we refer to as a woman's menses or period.

In the pre-menopausal years leading up to the menopause transition a woman will probably notice a change in the frequency, heaviness or lightness of her periods as the balance of hormones in her body changes. During the menopause transition itself these periods gradually become more and more erratic. A woman is said to be post-menopausal when she has not had menstrual bleeding for 12 months. So the menopause is a gradual process. The transition from being a woman capable of reproduction to being a woman beyond her reproductive years usually happens over a period of six to ten years. It is not an illness but simply a consequence of biological ageing.

In some countries and cultures it is a time of a woman's life which people celebrate; a mature woman has wisdom and life experience which she can use to help others. Before contraception became common practice many women may well have looked forward to the arrival of the menopause to escape from the relentless cycle of pregnancy, birth and child rearing.

Physical symptoms associated with the menopause

For some women, the accompanying signs and effects that can occur during the menopause transition years may interfere with their daily activities and affect their sense of well-being. Most women find that they simply feel more tired than before. Women of this age group are often trying to juggle work, their teenage children and ageing parents in this part of their lives.

Other common physical features of the menopause are hot flushes, vaginal dryness, joint pain, heart palpitations and dryer skin that is less elastic than before. Some menopausal women experience insomnia and difficulty with sleeping. Migraines, mild incontinence or frequent urination can also occur. Not everybody will suffer from any or all of these symptoms.

Feeling comfortable during the menopause

If you are beginning to experience the onset of the menopause then following the sensible advice already given in this book about diet, exercise, sleep and relaxation will help.

On a practical level, choosing clothes that are not too tight and are made from natural fibres can help to make hot flushes more bearable. Learn to dress in easy-to-take-off layers and switch to stockings instead of tights which are much healthier anyway! If you are going to be in a hot room, take a fan (traditional or battery operated) with you.

You might like to wear your hair up or tied back from your face if it is long or at least have a clip or hair elastic handy for hot moments!

Avoid heavy make-up which will streak if you break out in a sweat. Ask a make-up professional to advise you on products for your age group. Do drink plenty of water throughout the day to keep yourself hydrated.

Emotions

Some women experience emotional and psychological issues such as depression, mood swings and anxiety, perhaps for the first time in their lives. They may feel less attractive than before, comparing themselves unfavourably with younger women. Our emotional reaction to the menopause may depend a great deal on our personalities and how happy we already feel in our personal life.

This book already encourages readers to get out in the fresh air, take exercise and pursue hobbies to maintain a positive outlook. However, do not be afraid to ask for medical help if you think that you might be suffering from depression or anxiety at this time. Your doctor may advise a course of anti-depressants in conjunction with counselling.

Hormone Replacement Therapy

Your doctor may also suggest hormone replacement therapy or HRT. This treatment consists of oestrogen and progesterone for a woman who has an intact uterus, or oestrogen alone for a woman who has had a hysterectomy. The oestrogen can be taken from the urine of pregnant horses or made from plants while the progesterone is made synthetically and is known as progestogen. There are over fifty different types of HRT currently available and your doctor will send you to a menopause specialist to establish the correct treatment for you. Traditionally such therapy was provided as tablets but it is now available as skin patches, gels, skin sprays and implants just under the skin.

The NHS Choices website (UK) gives the benefits of HRT as the following: "relief from hot flushes, less vaginal dryness, bladder leaks and recurrent urinary tract infections, a better sex drive, reduced risk of bone fractures associated with osteoporosis and a reduced risk of bowel cancer." The website also states that the use of HRT "slightly raises your chance of developing the following conditions: breast cancer, ovarian cancer, blood clots, deep vein thrombosis or suffering a stroke...Most experts now agree that if HRT is used on a short-term basis for no more than five years, the benefits outweigh any risks."

The menopause is a significant time in any woman's life. Make sure that you take full advantage of preventative medical care such as mammograms for the early detection of breast cancer and smear tests to check for cervical cancer. To ensure good physical and mental health in later life it is also important that we ask for help with managing the symptoms of the menopause when this becomes necessary. Try to put your own needs first for at least part of everyday and part of every week so that you continue to enjoy life and feel good.

Can cosmetic surgery help my body look younger and feel better?

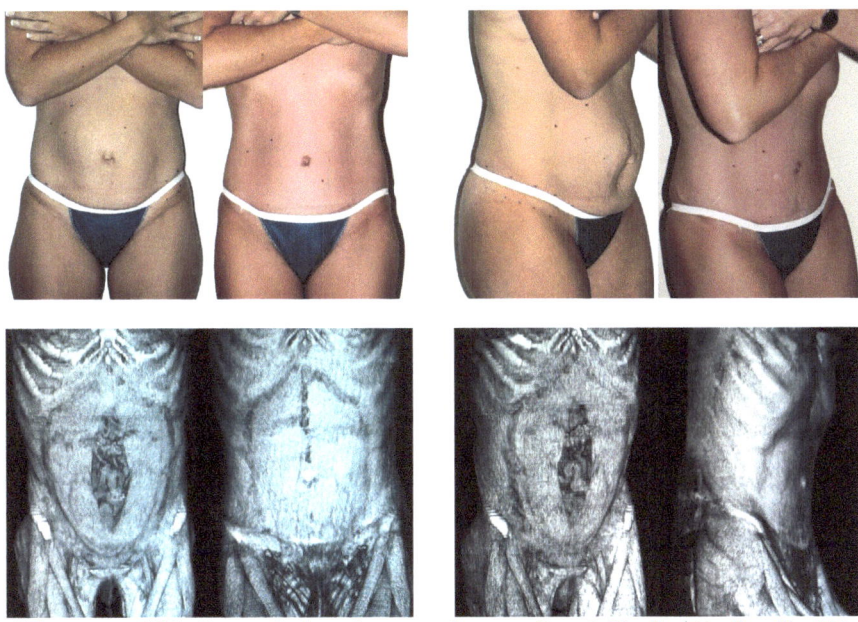

"Tummy tuck" before and after photos and scans, Otto J. Placik / Emilymiller123

Some people will never need cosmetic surgery or even consider it as an option. They were slim, active and healthy as children and young adults. They continue to exercise well into middle age and beyond. They keep active and have a good body image. They accept the signs of ageing with confidence and *joie de vivre*.

Other people are not so lucky. Perhaps illness, lack of incentive to exercise or a poor diet when young caused problems such as weight gain and low self-esteem: "I'm not very good at sport so I'll avoid it at all costs". Cosmetic surgery procedures to correct sagging skin after significant weight loss in women usually involve tummy tucks, breast lifting and sometimes liposuction. This drastic surgery often requires the surgeon to create a new belly button or new nipples for the patient. Women with very large busts may opt for a breast reduction to ease the strain on their backs and necks. They might also take this course of action to make exercising more comfortable.

There is also the question of gravity and the loss of collagen as we age which makes skin sag and makes our bodies look older. We can help ourselves to maintain a healthy figure and skin tone by avoiding drastic weight gain or weight loss. It may seem like stating the obvious but eating healthily throughout your life, exercising and avoiding smoking are better than relying on cosmetic surgery.

After pregnancy and childbirth

In an ideal world we'd all have time to go to the gym and go for lovely long walks at the weekend. For many women the crunch time with their bodies comes after pregnancy. We are so caught up with babies and children that there is little time or energy to exercise in the ways we did before having a family. So we have to be clever and get our exercise running after the little darlings in the park, or pop them in the pushchair and get out of the house for a walk at least once a day, rain or shine!

Some women find it difficult to lose that "mummy tummy" despite exercising, stomach crunches and sensible eating. Let's face it, the skin of the abdomen has been stretched out of all proportion as have the layers of muscle and soft tissue underneath. After a second, third or fourth child this becomes even more obvious with some women, while others seem genetically pre-disposed to snap back into shape. Women who have undergone a caesarean birth are advised not to exercise for a good few months after the operation and may find that the scar causes discomfort when they do resume. It can be ever so irritating when people look at your belly and say "Oh are you pregnant again?" when in fact through no fault of your own you just have naturally slacker skin and muscle!

If a tummy tuck or abdominoplasty gives a woman confidence to feel good about herself and her body again then the procedure is well worth the money and the effort. The surgery involves the removal of excess skin and fat from the middle and lower abdomen in order to tighten the muscle and fascia of the abdominal wall. It is not to be undertaken lightly as the initial recovery time is up to four weeks, depending on the particular type of abdominoplasty performed. Patients usually wear a surgical support corset during this time to help to support the affected muscles and they also refrain from heavy activity. Full recovery takes place within the next three to six months and the scars will continue to fade after that time.

Will this kind of procedure ultimately help a woman look younger and feel better? The evidence suggests that it will help some women. Modern women need to be active, fit, healthy and confident to deal with the everyday demands of work, home, relationships and family.

Breast lifts or augmentation

Other surgery which can form part of a "mummy makeover" is a breast lift. The most common breast lift operation, called mastopexy, repositions the nipple higher on the chest wall. Women can have this procedure as an out-patient, i.e., without an overnight stay in hospital if all goes well. It takes about three hours and is usually done under a general anaesthetic. The surgeon removes extra skin and lifts the breast tissue up into the correct location. Some women also get breast implants at the same time as their breast lift. The surgeon inserts the implants and then closes and bandages the breasts. Often tiny drains are put into the breasts for 24 to 48 hours. The disadvantages of this sort of surgery can be scarring and sometimes infections.

If you have just had a baby it is usual for your breasts to feel very much smaller and rather like empty sacks after you finish breast-feeding. Don't immediately despair and ring the nearest plastic surgeon. As your hormones get back to normal, so long as you eat healthily and take light exercise, you will probably find that your bust fills out again. Some brand new properly fitting bras with adequate support are essential at this stage of your life. Opt for swimwear with support also; halter neck styles and under-wiring work well.

You can have a breast lift at any age after your breasts have finished developing. You may also have one before or after you are pregnant. You should still be able to breast feed after a breast lift.

Cosmetic surgery following a medical procedure

Statistics suggest that one in eight women will suffer from breast cancer during their lives, based on a population that lives to the age of seventy. Breast re-construction is often chosen by women who have had a breast or both breasts removed while being treated for cancer. The breast is rebuilt either during the mastectomy operation or afterwards. This may be done by using either an implant or tissue from another part of the patient's body or a combination of both. Usually the shape of the breast is established first and then the new nipple and its surrounding areole are added in a later operation.

You may feel after reading the paragraph above that you can live with your slightly sagging but healthy breasts after all.

Facelifts

A facelift or rhytidectomy is a surgical procedure carried out by a plastic surgeon with the aim of rejuvenating a patient's face. As we age many of us experience sagging skin, increasingly hollow cheeks and a loss of definition around the chin and neck. Some people are bothered by this and opt for surgery. Other people simply don't care and are quite happy with the signs of ageing.

Plastic surgery is expensive and painful, usually requiring a general anaesthetic or sedation. There are risks of infection or a poor result and often the recovery time is quite long (six weeks and more to be back to normal). However some people feel that the end result is worth the effort.

Most plastic surgeons practise various different types of facelift surgery. At a consultation the procedure with the best outcome is chosen for each patient. The patient's expectations, their age, possible recovery time and areas to improve are some of the many factors taken in consideration before choosing a particular type of facelift.

In a traditional facelift, an incision is made in front of the ear extending up into the hairline. The incision curves around the bottom of the ear and then behind it, usually ending close to the hairline on the back of the neck. After the skin incision is made, the skin is separated from the deeper tissues with a scalpel or scissors over the cheeks and neck. The deeper tissues or SMAS, the fascial suspension system of the face, can be tightened with sutures, with or without removing some of the excess deeper tissues. The skin is then redraped and the surgeon decides how much excess skin to remove. The skin incisions are closed with sutures and staples.

A Mid Facelift is often suggested to people in their forties who don't yet need a neck lift but wish to deal with sagging cheeks and nose-to-mouth lines. The surgeon makes several small incisions along the hairline and inside the mouth, this way the fatty tissue layers can be lifted and repositioned with very few visible scars. This improves the nose-to-mouth lines and the roundness over the cheekbones. The recovery time is quite short and this procedure is often combined with a blepharoplasty (eyelid surgery).

The Thread Lift or Feather Lift is a less invasive surgical option, which is often used for people who seek minor improvements to treat sagging around the eye, forehead, and nasolabial fold areas. The lift can be performed under local anaesthetic and the surgeon uses a barb suture technique. The threads that hold the skin into place do not dissolve but remain in place, keeping the lift in effect, as no skin is cut away. The long term effects of this procedure are less aesthetically pleasing than other surgical options.

A Subperiosteal Facelift is done by vertically lifting the soft tissues of the face, completely separating it from the underlying facial bones and elevating it to a more aesthetically pleasing position. This corrects deep nasolabial folds and sagging cheeks. The technique is often combined with standard techniques, which provide a long-lasting rejuvenation of the face and is done in all age groups. The difference between this and other lifts is that the Subperiosteal Facelift has a longer period of facial swelling after the procedure.

As you might expect with a Skin-Only Facelift just the skin of the face is lifted and not the underlying SMAS, muscles or other structures. This is not a long lasting solution; usually the lift re-sags within 6 to 12 months after the procedure. A Skin-Only Facelift is only considered because it has fewer complications and is not as technically demanding as the SMAS or other types of lifts.

The MACS Facelift (Minimal Access Cranial Suspension) corrects sagging facial features through a minimal incision, lifting them vertically. There are many advantages to having a MACS Facelift rather than a traditional facelift. The MACS Facelift leaves a smaller scar in front of the ear, instead of behind, which is much easier to hide. Overall, this facelift is safer because less skin is raised. There is a reduced risk of bleeding and nerve damage. The operation is also quicker; 2.5 hours instead of the 3.5 hours that a traditional facelift requires. The recovery period is also shorter; 2–3 weeks instead of 3–4 weeks. Most importantly the results of the MACS Facelift are considered to be very natural.

Temporary cosmetic facial procedures

Common sense should tell us that Botox and fillers are last resorts. Do you really want to put yourself through a fair amount of pain and risk unpleasant side effects? Do you want a forehead that doesn't move? Would it not be better to eat well, take exercise, avoid smoking, excessive drinking and over exposure to UV rays? Some of us have probably become conditioned by TV and women's magazines where celebrity women, who depend on "their looks" to keep their career going end up looking a bit plastic.

Injectable fillers

Also known as dermal or soft-tissue fillers, these treatments can improve the appearance of ageing skin by filling in the area underneath it. Some injectable fillers are "natural" and some are synthetic. They are used to smooth out wrinkles, fine lines and deep creases, fill out thin or wrinkled lips and plump up cheeks. They can also help to contour the jaw line and other areas of the face.

Hyaluronan (hyaluronic acid) is a common ingredient in injectable fillers such Juvederm and Restylane. Results last for six months or maybe longer, depending on the individual patient, the skill of the doctor who administered the treatment and the type of filler. As with all medical or cosmetic procedures one should be aware of possible unpleasant side effects, such as swelling, redness and bumps or nodules under the skin where the filler has been injected.

Botox

Popularly known by its trade name, Botox, botulinum toxin is used in small doses for various cosmetic and medical procedures. Rather than "filling" a wrinkle, Botox relaxes the muscle underneath it. In cosmetic treatments it is often used to temporarily diminish lines on the forehead or between the eyebrows to give the face a more "relaxed" look. Results tend to last between six weeks and eight months.

Botulinum toxin is in fact a protein and neurotoxin produced by the bacterium clostridium botulinum. It is the most acutely toxic substance known to us; in humans a lethal dose is 1.3–2.1 ng/kg administered intravenously or intramuscularly and 10–13 ng/kg when inhaled. Botulinum toxin can cause botulism, a serious and life-threatening illness in humans and animals.

Fillers and Botox should always be administered by a registered, qualified practitioner. Unpleasant side effects of the treatment, which are generally minor and temporary, can be paralysis of the wrong muscle group and/ or an allergic reaction. Bruising at the site of injection is not a side effect not of the toxin, but rather the mode of administration. Some Botox users have suffered drooping eyelid(s), double vision, slight facial paralysis or have been unable to close their eyes after treatment. Apparently this wears off in around six weeks.

In the long term the continued use of Botox may cause deterioration in the muscles of a person's face around the area treated simply because that person is not exercising the face in a normal way. Some scientists claim that being less able to express emotions facially is damaging for the human brain also. All this is certainly food for thought.

Is it worth it?

It would be wonderful to think that we lived in a society where age, wisdom and laughter lines were celebrated. Have we ever undermined somebody's confidence by making unkind remarks about their appearance? Unfortunately in the western world too many people are under pressure to compete in the job market where youth is sometimes valued over experience. Perhaps we should address those issues that make us frown or our lifestyles, rather than resorting to quick fix Botox or the knife.

It is obvious that nobody should commit themselves to cosmetic surgery without researching the facts. If we choose to have a cosmetic procedure are we doing it for ourselves or to please other people? If you are considering cosmetic surgery you need to be honest with yourself about your expectations. However, we should bear in mind that everyone is different and we are all entitled to our own opinions.

And finally...

If all your attempts to keep looking and feeling young the sensible way are not sufficient here are some extra (tongue in cheek) tips:

Only hang out with friends who are older than you, or look older.

Wear sunglasses when you go out in daylight.

Select bars and restaurants with low lighting when you go out with friends or on dates. Avoid venues with bright or fluorescent lighting.

Think twice before getting yourself a toy boy – he might be fun for a while but you may end up looking older by comparison and therefore somewhat 'cougarish'.

Instead acquire a boyfriend, partner or husband who is definitely at least ten years older than you. If you're single and feeling cheeky how about hiring a "mature but dashing" escort for special occasions?

Conclusion

I hope that I have shown in this book that there are small things that we can do every day or every week to look after our health and to make ourselves feel better.

Having researched the sections on cosmetic surgery I know that personally I would do quite a lot to avoid having to resort to these procedures. I also realised that most of the women that I think look great, i.e. comfortable in their own skins, benefit from a positive outlook on life.

We cannot predict what life will throw at us in terms of health and relationships but we can eat well and exercise appropriately. If we avoid smoking and excessive sun exposure we give ourselves the best chance of looking good in our forties, fifties and beyond.

Acknowledgements

With grateful thanks to:

Linda, Denise, Elizabeth, Penny, Maria, Gail, Rowena, Clare, Catherine, Susan, Sonja, Mia, Carolyn, Lisa, Anna Karin, Pippa, Kim, Patricia and Madeline.

Also to Larry Davids for the idea and to Rick Lomas for the technology!

Ilustrations

All photographs by Susan Lomas except:

P. 37 Photograph of Lisa Lams by Anna Karin Heedh. Jewellery by Stella & Dot.

P. 31 Detail of cover photograph.

Susan Lomas

About the author

Susan Lomas (née Clements) was born in Watford, England in 1964. Rather an energetic child, she studied ballet for a while, quickly moving on to ballroom and Latin American dancing. She was educated in north London and gained a BA Honours degree in Fine Art Painting at Norwich School of Art in 1986. Susan taught Art and Design in a number of schools in Hertfordshire and Buckinghamshire during the 1980s and 1990s. She found that aerobics, yoga and swimming were excellent ways of keeping fit and coping with the demands of a teaching career. She also decided to buy a motorbike and obtain her motorbike licence so she could zoom around the countryside more easily.

In 2001 Susan decided to explore the southern French Alps and ended up making her home there. Her main passions in life continue to be Art, Literature and Music. Susan's outdoor pursuits are landscape photography, hiking in the mountains and skiing. In 2012 she published a book entitled "The History of Serre Chevalier and Briançon" which was the first detailed history of her adopted French valley written in English. She has also produced a series of watercolours depicting scenes from the Serre Chevalier valley.

Susan is a firm believer in the creative process. Like many other artists or writers she has found that an idea for a book or painting often suggests or imposes itself. She enjoys the challenge of bringing the idea to life and communicating it to others.

SusanLomas.com